LIVE LIFE PAIN FREE

Live Life Pain Free

Book design by:
Arbor Books, Inc.
www.arborservices.co

Printed in the United States of America

Live Life Pain Free
Dr. Hazmer Cassim

1.Title 2. Author 3. Therapy

Library of Congress Control Number: 2016914941
ISBN: 978-0-692-77942-2

LIVE LIFE PAIN FREE

By

Dr. Hazmer Cassim

Pain Management Physician

Dedication

It is the mind, that confuses the heart.
Deep down one always knows the truth, but the mind convinces one, of what must be done. In the silence of thought, however one can achieve this plane of being, the sound of a heart's desire, echoes beyond reason and logic, to express truth.
Listen, you will hear.
Believe and you can be.
Pause and you can experience.
Life is fleeting.
Moments are- F O R E V E R

To my parents Fameeda and Haniffa for unconditional love.
To my sister Fahma, my roomie, my buddy, my pal.

To my family and friends, for being the rainbows and flowers in this field of life.

To my patients, for teaching me that being a good physician begins with being a kind person.

Special thanks to Deb DeSantis and Kevin Holland for helping me edit this book

Table of Contents

Introduction

There were many reasons why I decided to spend my life helping people cope with pain. One of the most important was family.

My grandfather lived in Sri Lanka, then known as Ceylon, in the 1940's and had served in World War II under the British flag. Returning home after the war, he began practicing medicine at the same time the nation was proclaiming its independence from the British Empire. He spent the remainder of his life treating the local villagers. There were, in fact, a number of doctors in my family: my father, my uncle, and my two cousins. I remember watching with fascination as my grandfather, father, and other relatives treated people. In other countries, I'm sure that famous athletes and musicians were the heroes of children my age, but the people I most admired saved lives.

While she wasn't a doctor, my grandmother also showed me the importance of the medical profession in a different way. When I was very young, I would often spend time with my grandparents. I remember many times when I would wake in the middle of the night to the sound of raindrops on the roof. Despite waking me, I never found the rain disturbing. Quite the contrary, I found it peaceful, calming, and almost musical. I remember going to the window on those nights to watch the rain fall. My grandmother, who was no doubt roused by the same sound, would often stand beside me and watch as well. After all these years, I still treasure those memories. Unfortunately, I don't have nearly as many such memories as I would like, because when I was still young, my grandmother developed breast cancer.

It was at this point that I realized, doctors could not cure every affliction, nor save every life. There was nothing that medical science, or more specifically the medical science available at that time in Sri Lanka, could do to save my grandmother. I remember watching her slow struggle with an affliction that still claims thousands of lives every year. Today, there are a number of treatments that might have saved her life, but at the time, there wasn't much that medical technology could do for her. There are also a number of methods that could have at least helped her cope with the pain as she struggled, but back then she was simply given Tylenol every six hours, which did nothing for her.

I suppose we all hope that, when we finally die, it will be peacefully in our sleep. But the sad truth is that, for many of us, death is a slow and painful process. Far from resenting the doctors who couldn't help my grandmother, watching her struggle simply crystallized my admiration for the men and women who dedicated their lives to helping the sick. The experience also served to remind me that medical science still had, and still has, many unexplored areas worthy of investigation. Even if we can't cure every illness or heal every injury, I believe we can do far more to relieve pain, especially the long-term pain that accompanies so many medical conditions.

Of course, pain isn't only a symptom of fatal conditions. In fact, coping with some amount of pain is part of dealing with just about any medical condition, from a sprained wrist to cancer. Oftentimes, pain is the first symptom we notice of a more serious condition and, too often, we choose to ignore it as "just some minor ache" until the underlying cause becomes more serious.

Choosing Pain Management

My family moved to the United States when I was a teenager, and it was during my time at the University of Texas at Austin that I decided to pursue a degree in medicine. The fact that so many of my family members were physicians was one reason for the decision.

Choosing to pursue medicine was hardly the last important decision I had to make when attending college. There was also the question of what I would choose as a specialty. Initially I considered pediatrics, because I enjoyed the idea of working with children. I also considered specializing in radiology, like my uncle. Eventually, I decided to specialize in pain management, specifically physical medicine and rehabilitation with a subspecialty of interventional pain management.

Memories of my grandmother suffering from pain that could have been better treated were certainly part of what brought me to this decision. But I was also excited by the new frontiers that pain management research had to offer. Pain management methods can be crude in a third-world country, like my home in Sri Lanka, but I was surprised to find that, even in the United States of America, there wasn't nearly enough being done to treat those suffering in pain.

This is not to say that I was alone in seeing pain management as an unexplored frontier. I had several instructors, whom I consider to be mentors, who helped me understand how much more could be done for pain management. Two men in particular had a strong influence on me during my studies. Rather than run down a list of titles and credentials for each of them, I'll just call them Dr. Miles and Dr. David, each of whom influenced my studies and how I would eventually apply those studies in different ways.

Dr. Miles taught me how to listen to a patient. For most people, listening seems like a simple enough skill. It is not. It can grow even more difficult the longer you practice, as you're tempted to adopt a "seen it all before" attitude and assume you know what a patient is going to tell you before he or she even walks into your office. Truly listening to a patient means approaching each of them as a blank slate, not projecting a diagnosis just because one patient superficially reminds you of another. When you're dealing with any specialized form of medicine, it can be tempting to simply repeat the same diagnosis over and over again, whether or not it's relevant to a specific individual.

For instance, when I am consulted to help a person, and meet them for the first time, I have already read their information, reviewed their X-ray and MRIs, and I have a good impression of the problem. But, it is only after talking, evaluating and really listening to a patient that I come up with a solution to help them.

On the other hand, it's important when listening to distinguish between a patient listing symptoms and simply giving a self-diagnosis. Much like a doctor who's grown too accustomed to treating the same condition repeatedly, a patient who's dealt with pain symptoms over an extended period of time is bound to come up with theories about the source of those symptoms. Those theories can become convictions before he or she ever sets foot in a doctor's office. This problem grows worse with the various websites that are meant to provide patients with important medical information but can be misused as diagnostic tools. In a way, active listening involves doctors learning to disregard their own preconceived notions, as well as the preconceived notions of their patients.

Dr. David focused more on honing my technical skills, specifically regarding advanced procedures such as intrathecal therapy (delivering pain medication to the spinal fluid for more effective treatment) and kyphoplasty (surgically filling in the damaged or collapsed vertebrae in order to restore the proper shape of the spinal column). He even taught me the best way to perform advanced spinal injections by learning how to place the injection at the best location, using the appropriate level of anesthesia. In so doing, it was possible to perform a nearly painless epidural, which can, if done incorrectly, be extremely painful. While Dr. Miles taught me how to gather useful information from what a patient told me, Dr. David's training was more concerned with evidence-based medicine. Simply put, Dr. Miles helped me develop a discerning ear, while Dr. David helped me develop a discerning eye.

Patients can certainly speak to how they feel and what symptoms they're experiencing, but not all of the symptoms they exhibit will be immediately evident to them. For example, muscle tone can be an indicator of actual pain levels, and a change in posture is often a good indicator that muscles have become too tense, perhaps slowly over a long period of time. Another symptom that most patients are unlikely to notice is a loss of vibration sensitivity, which is one of the early signs of nerve damage. While most people only associate tuning forks with hearing tests, I was taught to always keep one handy when testing for nerve damage. Of course, the most significant symptom in determining whether pain is acute or chronic is simply the length of time that a patient has felt pain; even if that pain feels mild, it could be indicative of a significant problem if it's persistent for more than a few weeks.

In the end, I learned that effective pain management begins by building a trust between doctor and patient, where both learn to put aside preconceived notions and actively listen to one another in order to reach an accurate diagnosis. I've since treated thousands of patients suffering from chronic pain, and a significant part of my work involves educating them on the various treatments available to them. This book is intended as a guide to provide that education to anyone suffering from or treating chronic pain.

The Problems of Dealing with Pain Management

When we slam a knee into a table, catch a finger in a closing car door, knock our head in a low doorway, or have some other everyday accident, most of us will initially assume that the pain is temporary. We might assume that we can "walk it off," "sleep it off," "stretch it out," or "take a little something for it." We might try exercise, which may make the underlying injury that caused the pain even worse. We might try taking an aspirin, which may dull the pain while neglecting the underlying cause. We might even try alcohol or illegal drugs to numb the pain, which may, obviously, lead to even bigger problems like addiction. And the truth is that sometimes the pain does go away after a day or two, even if we do nothing about it. But sometimes that pain persists, getting gradually worse until we know that there's something seriously wrong.

On the other hand, there isn't always an obvious injury to indicate the source of pain. Sometimes we just wake up one day and feel bad. It could be a muscle ache or a stomachache or a headache. Maybe we tell ourselves that we slept badly, but again, if the pain persists, we eventually realize that the pain is a symptom of some larger problem. That's when many of us decide to consult with a physician, and that's when we run into one of the first great obstacles in diagnosing pain: a doctor's assumptions.

In cases when a patient reports feeling pain that has no obvious source, some doctors will be tempted to assume that the pain isn't real. With no overt symptoms and only the patient's description of how he or she feels, it's easy to dismiss pain sensations as exaggerations or outright lies. Of course, doctors aren't the only ones who have dismissed someone complaining about a mysterious pain. Don't you have a friend who's always complaining about this or that ailment, who always seems to be suffering from some vaguely understood condition? You're probably tempted to dismiss anything that person says with a statement like, "Oh, he's always complaining about something," or "It's probably all in her head." After a doctor has encountered a few cases of genuine hypochondria, reports of pain without overt symptoms will likely be viewed with at least some suspicion.

Sometimes a patient genuinely isn't feeling any pain and is simply reporting false symptoms in an attempt to get a prescription for painkillers. One of the warning signs that a patient is reporting false symptoms is if he or she asks for a specific drug instead of simply stating the symptoms and waiting for a diagnosis. OxyContin is one of the most popular "requested" drugs, along with oxycodone, Percocet, Vicodin, and morphine. Sometimes, the patients are looking for drugs to feed an addiction; however, they can also be attempting to acquire drugs to sell.

Early in my medical training I met Faye. Faye was a very sweet 68 year -old woman who had a long history of low back pain. Her primary care doctor wanted me to help, because Faye was using very high dosages of pain medication, specifically OxyContin, four to five times a day. However, she still had pain that was not improving. When I first met Faye, I reviewed her MRI and spoke to her about a treatment plan. Over the course of the next six months we worked together using multiple treatments the helped to improve her back pain. Faye never missed an appointment, she was always punctual and loved to smile. She was a very interesting woman who had travelled the world and would share pictures of the many fascinating cities she had visited in her life. But I noticed no matter what we tried, Faye needed more OxyContin. It was later that winter in Minneapolis, when two officers of the DEA (Drug Enforcement Administration) visited my office. They had been investigating Faye. I was shocked to realize that she had been getting OxyContin from multiple physicians in the area and selling the pills for a significant profit. Later that day I tried calling Faye, but her home and cell phone were disconnected. I was disappointed to learn that Faye had deceived me.

Doctors who prescribe painkillers for patients they know (or simply suspect) are faking symptoms can face severe legal penalties. Even physicians who give a diagnosis based on false information that they believed at the time to be true, can be held accountable if it's obvious that they didn't make a sufficient effort to determine whether or not a patient was being honest about his or her pain symptoms. Each physician has to rely on his or her own experience and trained perception to determine the honesty of a patient.

Like most people who become doctors, I pursued this profession out of a desire to help people, and like most doctors, I've had to deal with patients who are exaggerating, if not completely making up, pain symptoms. This balancing act, between taking a patient's account seriously and understanding that self-diagnosis is often inaccurate, is one of the most important skills a doctor has to develop. It's part of the listening skills I learned though my years of training in medicine. Speaking personally, I will say that if I ever do make a mistake, it will be in favor of taking the patient at his or her word, rather than assuming that they're exaggerating or lying. In the end, trusting the patient has to be a priority, even with the risks it brings.

Determining whether or not the pain a patient describes is genuine isn't the only challenge in making a diagnosis. There's also the question of whether that pain is acute or chronic. Quite simply, acute pain is short term, while chronic pain is long term (over 3 months, technically speaking). For patients suffering from acute pain, there are a number of effective treatments that have been around for quite some time. With chronic pain, however, the treatments become more complicated than simply prescribing drugs, which is not to say that prescribing drugs isn't often a part of such treatment.

For a long time, the methods for treating chronic pain were identical to the methods used for treating acute pain. My grandmother was given the same medicine for cancer that someone might be given for a bad headache. Even if she had been living in the United States at that time, morphine or other drugs that she would have been given wouldn't have been enough to help her effectively deal with chronic pain. The problem with most forms of pain medication is that they were not originally developed for long-term usage. Eventually, a patient can develop a tolerance for many drugs, at which point doctors will likely react by simply raising the dosage. This pattern of increasing dosage taking place over an indefinite period of time can eventually result in a patient becoming addicted or, at the least, suffering from various severe side effects.

Take a minute to consider those who suffer from addiction. Chances are, some of them suffer from addiction to illegal drugs such as cocaine or heroin, but addiction can as easily occur with doctor-prescribed painkillers. These "medical addictions" may start out differently than addictions to "street drugs," but the symptoms and difficulty in managing them are often the same. Addicts not only need the drug to continue with day-to-day activities, but they will need an ever-increasing amount of the drug, and the side effects will eventually make it impossible for them to even fake being "all right." In addition, once a physician realizes that the patient has become addicted, he or she will likely cease prescribing the medication entirely. Of course, a responsible physician will also take steps to help the patient deal with addiction, but doctors are limited in what they can make their patients do. Given the social stigma that accompanies drug addiction, many patients will refuse to even consider treatment, since that would mean admitting that they have an addiction. Without a legal source for the drug, many addicts will turn to illegal means to continue feeding their addictions.

Besides addiction, reliance on drugs alone for treating chronic pain fails to deal with the underlying cause of that pain. Issues like joint damage, nerve damage, and muscle tension and stress often require other forms of treatment to be properly resolved. All of this isn't to say that medication isn't an important part of treating chronic pain. It's just that chronic pain requires a far more comprehensive style of treatment, of which medication is only one important component.

The Comprehensive Approach to Chronic Pain Management

There is no single way to deal with chronic pain that works for everyone. Each patient needs to be considered as an individual with a unique set of symptoms and accompanying treatment needs. But even an individual suffering from pain symptoms shouldn't rely on only one method of treatment. The most effective chronic pain management strategy will require you to use several different methods simultaneously. If you're reading this book, chances are that you've been coping with chronic pain for some time before finally seeking help. And while your doctor certainly has a great deal of knowledge in dealing with chronic pain, he or she will likely be consulting with specialists for each method of treatment being used. Please keep in mind that the most important specialist that any doctor will consult in any diagnosis, is the patient. Nobody knows the symptoms you're suffering from better than you, and the key to effective comprehensive treatment is to keep yourself, your physician, and all of the consulting specialists informed about any changes in your condition.

When I mentioned my grandmother being treated with Tylenol every six hours for her pain, I didn't mean to imply that there was anything wrong with prescribing Tylenol. If she'd been in America, she would have been given morphine or a similar drug and, for the time, there would have been nothing inappropriate about such treatment either. The real problem is that prescribing any medication, should not be the sole method of pain management employed by the doctor treating cancer pain.

Even today, many physicians still have a tendency to write a prescription and send the patient on his or her way. We've all seen the commercials for various "miracle" drugs that promise to alleviate, if not completely eliminate, the pain that comes from various conditions. You might have noticed that these commercials often show men and women engaging in various physical activities—playing football, doing yard work, riding horses—with no apparent sign of pain. To say that these are actors who don't actually have the conditions these drugs are meant to treat should go without saying. But just as significantly, these commercials never show people engaging in physical therapy, undergoing surgery, reevaluating their diets, or going through any other sort of treatment, which no doubt leads many patients to believe that all they'll need to do to stop feeling pain is to get that miracle pill. Most of these commercials end with the suggestion to "ask your doctor if this drug is right for you." This is the opposite of how a consultation should go, with the patient not only determining his or her symptoms, but also making a diagnosis and deciding on the proper treatment without first consulting with a physician. This situation can be as difficult to handle as the drug addict reporting fake symptoms in order to get a prescription for narcotics. Unfortunately, some doctors will write such prescriptions based on nothing more than patient demand, and these physicians are rightly condemned by the larger medical community.

While proper medication is certainly one method of chronic pain management, it will only be fully effective if used in conjunction with other modalities. The five methods or pillars of chronic pain management that we'll be exploring are (1) medication, (2) behavior modification, (3) interventional therapy, (4) alternative treatments, and (5) physical rehabilitation. Again, none of these methods should be used on their own, and none of them should be considered the "most important" method. As we briefly review each method, please keep in mind that many books have been written and many courses taught on each of them. It is entirely possible for a doctor to devote his or her entire practice to any single one of these treatment methods, so please consider the following to be a series of introductions. After all these years, I'm still learning new things about pain management.

Medication

Medication is certainly not a recent innovation in pain management. Before there were physicians, as we would know them, pain was treated with a variety of herbal remedies. In fact, many deal with pain using "home remedies" or simply by having a few glasses of beer or some other alcoholic beverage. That's why having a couple of drinks or using some illegal narcotic like heroin to help cope with pain is often referred to as "self-medication." But for now, let's focus on the drugs that modern doctors traditionally use in pain management. These drugs can be broadly divided into two categories: opioid and non-opioid.

Opioid drugs, also known as narcotic drugs, are so named because they directly affect the opioid receptors in the brain or spinal column, essentially reducing or completely canceling pain signals so that the brain doesn't register them. If you're treating immediate pain resulting from, say, a broken limb, deep cut, or severe burn, opioid drugs can be extremely effective in numbing the affected area for a brief period of time (being an acute pain condition). During the first World War, many soldiers would carry injectable ampules of morphine as part of their military equipment; if they were injured on the field, they would take the morphine and go right back into battle. After the war, morphine (and various derivatives) was marketed as a miracle cure for all manner of pain. Without the proper understanding about the long-term side effects, morphine addiction became a widespread problem before the medical community and the government agreed that it needed to be regulated. These days, an increasing variety of opioid drugs are available, many tailored for specific effects. And while doctors receive much better training to minimize side effects, the possibility of side effects still exists.

As I said earlier, the most significant problem with prolonged usage of any opioid drug is that the body will build an increased tolerance with each dosage (as acute pain shifts to chronic pain), meaning that you'll need to administer a progressively larger dose to get the same effect each time. Sometimes, with increased dosage, the drug will begin to cause the pain that it was originally intended to alleviate; sadly, the reaction to this increase in pain is too often to simply increase the dosage further, which only exacerbates the problem. This condition, called opioid-induced hyperalgesia, is often not diagnosed. On the other hand, sometimes there is no ceiling to the effectiveness of some opioid drugs, meaning that you could theoretically continue getting the same results by administering an ever-increasing dosage indefinitely; however, other side effects to these drugs will grow worse over time. The worst side effect to most opioid drugs is the risk of becoming physically addicted, meaning that your body will continue to need the drug in order to function properly, even if you're no longer suffering from the pain symptoms that it was originally treating.

As I said, the list of available opioid drugs is extensive and includes buprenorphine (also known as Buprenex or Butrans), butorphanol, codeine, hydrocodone, hydromorphone (also known as Dilaudid, Exalgo, or Palladone), levorphanol (also known as Levo-Dromoran), meperidine (also known as Demerol), methadone (also known as Methadose, Diskets, or Dolophine), morphine (also known as Duramorph, DepoDur, Astramorph, or Infumorph), nalbuphine, oxycodone (also known as OxyContin, Roxicodone, or Oxecta), oxymorphone (also known as Opana), pentazocine (also known as Talwin), propoxyphene (also known as Darvon), and tapentadol (also known as Nucynta). Each of these drugs is used for pain conditions. Some of these cause side effects that can include headaches, difficulty in breathing, irregular heartbeat, constipation, dizziness, drowsiness, and nausea. Over time, these side effects can grow so intense that they may prove fatal. No matter what precautions you take, you need to understand that every single opioid drug, including everything listed here, can and has been abused. Ironically, some of these drugs were initially developed for the purpose of fighting addiction, by providing addicts with a substitute to help them wean themselves off the opioids to which they'd originally become addicted; these drugs include bupranorphine, methadone, and diamorphine (more commonly known as heroin) and have all, in turn, been abused.

Non-opioid drugs are distinguished from opioid drugs in that they do not work by reducing pain signals to the brain or spinal column. Instead, they effect a change at the source of the pain. For instance, a non-opioid drug might hinder the production of prostaglandins, a lipid compound that performs a variety of functions, such as sensitizing neurons to pain. Non-opioid drugs can also reduce inflammation of injured areas of the body, which in turn will reduce pain. Obviously, any such change in the body can have other side effects. Unlike opioid drugs, non-opioid drugs often do have a ceiling, meaning that there is a maximum dosage that, if exceeded, will produce no further positive effects. However, it should be noted that despite having a ceiling for their intended positive effects, the harmful side effects of non-opioid drugs still continue to increase with larger doses.

The most obvious advantage that non-opioid drugs have over opioid drugs is that non-opioid drugs are not physically addictive. This is not to say that non-opioid drugs can't be habit forming, but with these drugs the addiction will likely be psychological rather than physical. This is not to say that non-opioid drug addiction can't be just as problematic. In fact, part of the problem with psychological addiction is that, since patients are made aware that a non-opioid drug is not physically addictive, they might therefore consider it to be a "safe" drug and be less vigilant in maintaining the prescribed dosages. Some of the most commonly abused non-opioid drugs are muscle relaxants like cyclobenzaprine (also known as Flexeril) and carisoprodol (also known as Soma), as well as anticonvulsion drugs such as gabapentin (also known as Neurontin, Gralise, and Horizant).

Another key difference between opioid and non-opioid drugs has nothing to do with their chemical properties, but rather with their legal status. Many opioid drugs are regulated by the government, meaning that they are only available with a doctor's prescription. Other opioid drugs, such as heroin, are completely illegal. Non-opioids, on the other hand, are often far less regulated, and some are even available over-the-counter without a prescription. Again, this is not to say that there is no risk of abuse with non-opioids. You've no doubt noticed that even aspirin —perhaps the most common over-the-counter non-opioid available — comes in a bottle labeled with a series of warnings. However, since opioids are more heavily regulated and therefore harder to acquire, patients reporting fake symptoms are more likely going to do so in order to gain prescriptions for opioid drugs. It is also the reason why physicians are more reluctant to issue prescriptions for opioid drugs if there is any doubt about a patient's reported pain symptoms.

Some times, non-opioid drugs maybe more effective for specific types of pain. One common type of pain I see in patients is sciatica. Sciatica, clinically called radiculopathy, is a condition where nerves leaving the spinal cord, get trapped and become painful. This pain can even travel all the way down patients legs. A few years ago, I was sitting in a bus in London, going to visit some friends after I had attended a medical conference. A young man sat down next to me and was in obvious pain. He had difficulty bending his right leg and finding a comfortable position. After a few minutes of watching him I knew he had severe low back pain. After some time had passed, we started talking. He introduced himself as John. He was a new physician who had started working three months ago. He lived next to Greenwich Park in London, right next to the river Thames and took the bus to work daily. He had diagnosed himself with sciatica and was on his way to apply for time off work, because he could no longer sit or stand for very long and this made it difficult to treat patients. He was taking pain medication, but it was not helping. He had his MRIs with him and I took a look at the images. We spent the rest of the journey talking about what could be done for his pain so that he could continue to work. I recommended a non-opioid medication, gabapentin, which could help calm sciatica. At then end of the trip I wished him the best and we parted ways. John sent me an email many months later, thanking me for the suggestion.

Gabapentin had helped him more than the pain pills. I was happy that he was able to continue working as a physician.

Of course, physicians must always exercise caution when prescribing drugs, both opioid and non-opioid, for the treatment of chronic pain. In fact, it's not uncommon for physicians to administer one or more surveys to measure a patient's potential for addiction. The DIRE evaluation takes only a few minutes to administer and measures a patient's risk of addiction based on four factors: Diagnosis (how serious the pain condition is), Intractability (how committed the patient is to his or her own treatment), Risk (which is itself a combination of psychological, chemical health, reliability, and social support factors), and Efficacy Score (how effective drug treatments have been in the past). Another popular evaluation is the SOAPP (Screener and Opioid Assessment for Patients with Pain) evaluation, which is another brief test that measures a patient's history with drug use, as well as possible sources of stress and mood disorders. Obviously, these tests require honest input from the patients, which can be challenging to acquire at times.

While the effectiveness of both opioid and non-opioid drugs is well documented, the risk of addiction and other side effects only increases over time if both doctor and patient don't remain vigilant and honest with one another. This is why it's important for a doctor to maintain the same level of honesty that he or she expects from a patient, in order to build the trust necessary to continue comprehensive treatment.

Behavior Modification

One of the advantages to using a comprehensive treatment method for pain management is that it allows the patient to take a more active role in his or her treatment. And nowhere is that more apparent than in behavior modification. While medication treats pain directly (opioids shutting down pain signals to the brain and spinal column) and indirectly (non-opioids reducing the causes of pain, such as inflammation), it works on a strictly physical level. Simply put, you can take your medicine and immediately forget you've taken it, but the medicine will continue to work. Furthermore, medication often works in ways that you're unaware, such as harmful side effects.

With behavior modification, on the other hand, the patient is not only encouraged to be more aware of his or her pain and its underlying causes, but they'll monitor their pain in real time and take steps to consciously reduce it. Perhaps you're thinking this sort of treatment won't work on you; after all, if you could consciously reduce your pain, you'd already be doing it and wouldn't need to see a doctor at all. But in a way, reducing the pain is the easier part of behavior modification. The more difficult aspect is finding a way to accurately perceive the source of pain.

One process of behavior modification involves monitoring biofeedback. It begins with the patient being attached to a monitoring device. The sort of device being used depends on what involuntary process the doctor wishes to monitor. There are machines that monitor heart rate, sweating, brain wave activity, and skin temperature. Believe it or not, all of these bodily functions can, to some degree, be consciously controlled. However, when dealing with pain symptoms, you'll often use an electromyogram, which monitors muscle tension. The level of muscle tension is visually represented on a monitor so a patient can see the current level of tension he or she is experiencing. Alternatively, the tension could be represented by a tone that grows louder or softer, depending on the level of muscle tension. It's not uncommon for a patient to be surprised by the level of muscle tension his or her body is experiencing. Since tension can build in small increments over a long period of time, you may not be aware of how much tension your body is feeling; in effect, you slowly get used to the tension until you're no longer consciously aware of it, although you still feel its negative side effects.

Obviously, the next step of biofeedback treatment, once you're able to monitor your level of tension, is to consciously reduce that level. One of the easiest methods of accomplishing this relaxation is through slow, controlled breathing. Another method is to consciously flex a muscle, then relax it, over and over again, perhaps by bending a joint, gripping a rubber ball, or arching your back. Perhaps you will be asked to focus on a mental image or pleasant memory (a peaceful landscape or a vacation). You might be asked to perform a combination of these tasks. Whatever you do, you will be able to observe the change in your tension level on the monitor or hear it through a speaker. By experiencing tension through a sense other than touch, you can become truly aware of how tense your muscles have become and receive immediate feedback when the various relaxation methods have begun to work.

When you're starting out with biofeedback treatment, you'll likely need to visit your physician's office for each appointment. Typically most of us won't have the necessary monitoring devices at home, and you will want to have a doctor present, to guide you through the process and help if there are any problems. However, there are home-use versions of many of these devices, most of which can be hooked up to your personal computer, and in time your physician may decide that this is a viable alternative to regular office visits.

Obviously, there's only so much that can be accomplished in a single once-a-week visit with your physician. While biofeedback treatment can provide a surprising amount of stress and pain relief during that session, your stress and pain levels will likely rise back to their previous levels shortly after you leave the office. This is because many of us engage in lifestyle activities that put us at a higher risk for chronic pain. Perhaps we exercise too strenuously, don't get enough regular sleep, or engage in routine, nonpainful activities that nevertheless lead to pain-inducing conditions over time, such as frequent typing leading to carpal tunnel syndrome. Even your diet can affect pain symptoms. A once-a-week visit will not be enough to solve these problems, at least not in the long term, if not accompanied with other treatment methods. This is why there are also behavior modification treatment methods that take place outside of standard appointments, without a physician present.

An example of treatment that takes place largely outside of a physician's office is postural recognition. As stated earlier, bad posture can be the result of chronic pain. But bad posture can also be the cause of chronic pain. Postural recognition guides the patient through recognizing his or her own poor posture and then provides them with the steps necessary to begin correcting it. The process begins quite simply with the patient standing, sitting, and walking around the physician's office. The physician then guides the patient to assume a healthy posture during each of these activities. Of course, such treatments are meaningless if the patient simply goes back to assuming a poor posture once he or she leaves the doctor's office, so steps are also taken to help the patient keep track of his or her own posture throughout the day.

Since we all assume a natural, and often unhealthy, posture when we're not thinking about it, the patient is encouraged to set up an alarm that will go off every fifteen minutes as a reminder to check his or her posture. Eventually, the alarm will be reduced to perhaps once every two hours, then once a day, then once a week, until it can finally be discontinued altogether. Given that such frequent alarms can be disturbing to coworkers, family members, and anyone else sharing space with the patient, he or she might instead opt to place a visual marker— something as simple as a colored sticker—at a location that gets frequented throughout the day— the break room, the copy room, the bathroom, the kitchen, or some other location—so the patient has a reminder to check their posture every time they enter that room. Whatever reminder is used, eventually the patient will develop the unconscious habit of checking and adjusting their posture without needing reminders at all. This type of treatment can be highly effective when treating back or neck pain; however it is becoming more difficult for patients to receive health insurance coverage for postural recognition, since it's difficult to measure its effectiveness based solely on the office appointments.

While behavior modification often involves more effort (especially on the patient's part) than medication, there are certainly advantages to this method, chief among them being the lack of harmful side effects. This is not to say that harmful side effects aren't possible, but they tend to be more psychological than physical. As an example, if a patient enjoys a pastime that involves a lot of physical activity, such as golf, swimming, basketball, or hiking, some behavior modification treatments might hinder his or her ability to engage in such activity. It's like the old joke of a man telling the doctor, "It hurts when I do this," and the doctor's advice being simply, "Don't do that." Having to give up something that one enjoys doing due to pain treatment can lead to depression, which in turn can lead to other more overtly physical symptoms. In these cases, the solution is to find ways to modify how one engages in these pastimes so that muscle tension is lessened — modifying one's golf swing, using a different type of swimming stroke, or wearing a different pair of shoes. Alternatively, such pastimes can be used as a goal for behavior modification — reducing pain symptoms until the patient can enjoy these activities once again.

Behavior modification can also be the missing link to pain relief. It was my first summer in California, and I had completed a lecture in pain management for a conference in Palm Springs. That is where I met Jane. She was a 35 year-old lady who had debilitating neck pain for over ten years. She came to see me in my office a few weeks later and we discussed what I could do to help. She had tried many different treatments for her neck pain. Multiple physicians had worked on helping her. After reviewing all her records, medications, and multiple types of treatments, I concluded that over the past ten years she certainly had tried almost everything to help with her neck pain. We were both a bit disappointed that there was nothing more that could be done to help her. She was going to New Mexico to see her parents and I was going to think about what else could be done. As she was leaving my office, I noticed she had a large purse that she placed over one shoulder. It seemed she had been using that purse to carry her work documents for many years and was essential for her life style. Since I could not convince her to use a smaller purse, I told her to try behavior modification. She agreed to set her phone alarm to ring every 30 minutes for the first week. Each time the alarm rang she would move the purse to her other shoulder. My hope was, after a week she would no longer need the alarm to remind her to switch the purse to her other shoulder. About 7 months later I received a card from Jane. She was happy to be pain free. The alarm had been a reminder not only to her, but her co-workers as well, that her purse needed to be moved. Though she was not ready to down size her purse yet, she was doing well.

Since a patient can employ behavior modification techniques long after he or she has ceased seeing a doctor, such techniques are ideal for coping with long-term conditions. Such conditions require life-style changes that are more significant than simply remembering to take some pills once a day and therefore require a much greater commitment from the patient if they're going to work. For this reason, the treatments need to be easy to implement without additional medical equipment, easy to monitor, and conducive to a patient's lifestyle in both work and leisure activities.

Interventional Therapy

Sometimes, pain becomes so severe and unmanageable that a more direct method of treatment needs to be explored. Interventional therapy involves the physician performing one of several procedures to help alleviate pain, either by directly affecting the pain receptors or the cause of the pain. This treatment can involve something as simple as giving the patient an injection once every few months. It can also involve invasive surgery in the more extreme cases. While interventional therapy can certainly be part of a comprehensive treatment method, it's not an option employed without first giving a great deal of consideration.

When dealing with pain from an ongoing condition such as arthritis, the physician might administer an epidural injection of an anti-inflammatory medication, such as cortisone or steroids, at the source of the pain. Such injections have several advantages over more standard forms of administering medication. For one thing, the injections deliver therapeutic treatment right to the source of pain, rather than oral medication that has to go through the whole body. This direct delivery of treatment, which can send cortisone, heat, or electricity to the source of pain, can have a profound effect. Most of us have had inoculation shots administered at one time or another. You may have also donated blood or plasma at some point in your life. For that reason, you might believe that delivering an epidural injection is as simple as finding a vein and sticking in a needle. In practice, it's quite a bit more complicated.

The first epidural injections were administered in the 1920's and involved a far more haphazard process of trial and error. Generally, medical students learned how to properly give epidural injections by practicing on one another. Not only were the syringes poorly positioned, but the dosages were often decided by little more than guesswork and involved a variety of questionable drugs, including cocaine derivatives. Not only did this process result in many injuries, but it did not provide the students with adequate knowledge of how to safely administer such injections to their future patients.

Over time, epidural injections became more precise through the application of four different practices: (1) guided injections, (2) better training for physicians, (3) using a contrast liquid prior to injection, and (4) patient feedback. Starting in the 1950's, various scanning methods — X-rays/fluoroscope, CT-scans, ultrasound, and electromyography —were used to monitor the needle's position beneath the skin, in order to more accurately direct it. At the same time, physicians were better trained to recognize the anatomical landmarks that are necessary to precisely aim a syringe. A contrast liquid, such as iodine, would be initially injected near the nerve being treated in order to better highlight it under the fluoroscopic scanning device. Finally, patients were no longer given a general sedative, which would render them unconscious, during the procedure so they would be able to give their own feedback to aid the physician while he or she worked. By combining all of these practices, epidural injections became far safer and more effective for patients.

Once the physician is able to properly find the nerve, disc, or other target in need of treatment, there are several methods by which treatment can be administered. The most common method is to inject a combination of anti-inflammatory steroid (such as corticosteroid) and anesthetic directly around the spinal nerve in the epidural space. This type of epidural injection helps reduce inflammation which leads to the reduction, and potential resolution of pain. At times, pain medication such as fentanyl or morphine (opioids) are injected in the epidural space instead of anti inflammatory medication, this is helpful with childbirth or other events which can be acutely painful. Though both anti-inflammatory medication and opioids can be used in the epidural space at the same time, typically anti-inflammatory medication is reserved for pain conditions that are chronic.

In my practice interventional therapy is a very powerful method of pain relief. After initially discussing a treatment plan, interventional therapy is used to help not only treat, but also diagnose problems that are not easily identified in imaging (MRI, X- Ray, CT) and examination.

Pamela was a 56 year-old woman who had been dealing with neck pain for two years. She also had numbness and tingling in her right arm. Physical therapy and multiple medications had given her a little help. She came to see me with significant difficulty finding any position of comfort due to pain. She had been waking up every night due to numbness in her arm and was very frustrated since she no treatment had helped her this far. At our first meeting, we discussed a few short term strategies to give her comfort and I made some changes to her medication. I also ordered an MRI of her neck and she was to come see me to review the images and discuss a long-term solution to her pain. Neck or cervical MRI's allow physicians to see not only bones, like in X-rays, but also problems with the nerves, discs and even muscles. In Pamela's MRI, of the seven bones of her neck, there was a narrowing or stenosis of the spinal cord between cervical bone number 6 and 7 (stenosis of C6-C7).

This stenosis was squeezing the nerve going down her right arm causing not only neck pain, but also tingling, and numbness. This same scenario, known as sciatica, can occur in the low back or lumbar spine as well, where there are five bones numbered lumbar 1 though 5 (L1-L5). After discussing options Pamela and I decided to pursue an epidural steroid injection.

Pamela was a bit nervous on the day of the procedure as she had never had an epidural injection in her life. She could eat or drink anything she wanted and did not have any restriction. She could take all her usual medication, but had to stop any blood-thinning medication. I greeted Pamela when she arrived and the nurses took her blood pressure and asked her a few questions. We then took Pamela into the procedure room. Pamela laid facedown on a table, very similar to a massage table, with an opening for her face. I cleaned her neck with an alcohol-based cleaning solution . Then an x-ray machine was brought over her head. Using live X-rays, I saw the cervical 6 (C6) and cervical 7 (C7) bones. Then her skin was anesthetized and using live x-rays, I guided a needle between the bones and into the epidural space. The procedure can take anywhere from 5-15 minutes, but by using liberal amounts of anesthetic, Pamela was very comfortable. We kept talking about her visit to Venice beach throughout the procedure and she was pleasantly surprised when I said it was all done. She had about 50 percent reduction of pain immediately, but I did inform her that the medication I placed, an anti-inflammatory cortisone, a steroid known as Dexamethasone, can take up to seven days for full effect. Pamela continued to do well, she received one more injection a month later and when I saw her again her pain was well controlled. It has been two years now and Pamela is still doing well. She continues with her home exercises and is happy to get a full night's sleep without any pain.

Another method involves removing pain-causing nerves, rather then healing them with anti-inflammatory medication or numbing them with opioid medication. Removing nerves can be accomplished with chemicals and by freezing or heating them. Various chemicals, such as ethyl alcohol, or phenol, can be used to dissolve pain causing nerves in a process known as neurolysis. Freezing the neurons, is known as cryoablation and exposes nerves to extreme cold. Extreme heat can be used to burn the neurons by running an electrical current through them, this is known as radiofrequency lesioning.

Jason was an 85 year-old gentleman from south Florida with low back pain for over six months. He loved to play golf. But due to his back pain he had not been able to return to golf for the past five months and was depressed thinking his golfing days were over. He had completed physical therapy, home exercises and received multiple medications. He had even tried multiple epidural injections without much benefit. When I reviewed his MRI, even though there was stenosis, he also had a lot of arthritis know as spondylosis of the joints in his low back or lumbar spine. These small joints, the facet joints, can cause pain especially with movement. We discussed a few options and decided to pursue radiofreqency lesioning. Radiofrequency lesioning, also know as ablasion or rhizotomy, was the best option to dissolve the pain nerves (or medial branches), in Jason's back and give him relief for six months to two years. Jason did very well with the procedure. Two years later I saw Jason, on the Mission Hills golf course in Rancho Mirage. He had a big smile and a hug for me. He was still doing well, living life pain free.

Neuromodulation is another method of interventional treatment that physicians will recommend in more extreme cases of chronic pain. Quite simply, neuromodulation involves the insertion of a small electronic device, usually no larger than a quarter, beneath the skin. This device will remain in place for a long time, perhaps even permanently, and continue to help the patient cope with pain for several months, several years, or even for the rest of his or her life. This neuromodulation device can be placed on or near the spine, or on the area where the patient experiences pain. In any case, the device will aid in pain relief by either stimulating the nerve endings electronically or by injecting a small dosage of pain medication on a constant basis. Generally, the first neuromodulation procedure involves the physician inserting a temporary device beneath the skin in order to gauge its effectiveness; if benefit is present, it is replaced with a permanent version of the device. Since very low dosages are used for chemical neuromodulation in intrathecal therapy, the risk of addiction or other adverse side effects is greatly reduced. Adjustments to the device, changing batteries or refilling the medication, can be performed easily with a minimally invasive procedure. Dosage adjustments can be done through a remote control. In fact, these units have been in use since the 1960's to treat both acute and chronic pain. Today's technology has revolutionized the devices with increased sophistication of delivery and significant reduction in size. Unlike over-the-counter drugs, the potential to misuse such devices is minimal.

Maria is a 65 year-old woman who unfortunately had breast cancer which had spread or metastasized to her liver and bones. Though chemotherapy and radiation treatments had helped limit the spread of her disease, she was in severe pain. When cancer cells spread to the bone, it causes deep aching pain, that is very difficult to treat. Maria was on high dosages of pain medication that she took by mouth, as well as through her skin in the form of pain patches. She was also taking pain medication in the form of oral sprays. Even with such high dosages of medication, her pain had made her immobile and she had lost the will to move and stayed in bed most of the day. Also the side effects of the medication, worst of all the constipation, had become problematic. Shortly after I saw her in my office, her insurance company refused to pay for her pain medications. Despite all appeals, the insurance company refused to authorize the medication which gave Maria some comfort. This was a very difficult time and Maria's son was thinking the time had come to consider hospice, as Maria had lost her will to live. After a long discussion we decided to try an intra-thecal pain pump. This is a neuromodulation device that allows me to deliver pain medication directly to the spinal cord. It is a surgery that can take anywhere from 40 to 90 minutes. Maria was under general anesthesia, and I made a small opening in the middle of her back. Then I opened up the different layers of muscle and connective tissue until I came close to the spinal bones. Using a live x-ray, I guided a small tube into the spinal fluid sac, the thecal sac, around her spinal cord. Then I guided the tube, the catheter, along the spinal cord to the desired location. I connected this catheter underneath her skin and muscle to the reservoir, a hockey puck-shaped device. After making sure all connections were in place and verifying though infra-red connection that the reservoir was functioning, I closed all the incisions. The reservoir had morphine which was being delivered to Maria's spinal cord. This method of delivery now allows for very small dosages of medication, with less side effects and better pain control. Three hundred milligrams of oral morphine is equal to one milligram of morphine delivered in this intrathecal manner. After the surgery Maria no longer needed any pain medication. A few months ago, Maria and her son came to talk to all our staff at the spine and pain center. They wanted to thank our team for helping Maria become pain free. I was smiling looking at Maria, happy that she was doing so well. I also thought of my grandma. My grandma was five years younger than Maria when she passed from metastatic breast cancer. Sadly, she suffered in her final days. I wonder if she would have lived longer if her pain was under control. I will never know the answer, but I do know that many still suffer today, unaware of all the treatments available for pain. We must continue to educate the world on treatment options available to live life pain free.

Obviously, doctors are careful about recommending interventional therapy. The procedures generally don't take long, and recovery time, if any, is ordinarily quite brief. It can be an effective part of comprehensive treatment.

Alternative Treatments

Earlier, I mentioned how behavioral therapy methods might seem reminiscent of the stories you've heard about mystics using meditation to transcend pain. Such stories can give us a comical misunderstanding of such practices. A growing body of medical research shows many of these methods do work, although often for reasons other than what traditional practitioners may tell you.

You're no doubt familiar with acupuncture. Quite simply, acupuncture alleviates pain by applying pressure to precise points across the body. This pressure can be applied through small needles or simply by pressing down on the points with one's fingers, known as acupressure. According to many practitioners of this ancient healing art, the application of pressure allows the patient's life energy, known as "chi" or "qi", to flow more freely by breaking down blockages that exist between the body's twelve meridians. The pressure points don't always seem to connect intuitively with the pain points (for example, back pain might be alleviated by applying pressure to points on the ear), and there are a number of extremely complex and detailed charts depicting how various points on the body connect to various pressure points.

The more plausible medical explanation for acupuncture's effectiveness is that the application of needles or fingertip pressure releases the body's endorphins, which are a naturally occurring form of opiate that the body produces. Either way, acupuncture has been in use for over two thousand years, and its effectiveness has been well documented, even if the reason for said effectiveness is still open to debate.

Another alternative treatment method that is gaining medical credibility is hypnotherapy. Again, before you begin this type of treatment, you'll need to abandon the television sitcom image of the hypnosis stage acts you've probably seen where audience members are told to pretend they're chickens or other such silliness, or the man in a suit who waves a swinging watch in front of your face until you fall into a deep sleep. Basically, hypnosis involves a physician guiding a patient into achieving a more relaxed state using methods similar to what is used in the biofeedback method. Various medical studies conducted in recent years show that hypnosis can be effective in reducing pain symptoms for conditions ranging from cancer to fibromyalgia to arthritis. In addition, this form of treatment can be effective when dealing with psychological conditions, such as stress, that cause increased muscle tension, that in turn cause pain. Furthermore, these positive results come without the side effects that accompany medication.

Meditation is, in many ways, similar to hypnosis, in that it involves a largely self-induced state without needing medication or invasive surgery. The key difference between meditation and hypnosis is that meditation techniques are usually much easier for a patient to employ on his or her own, without needing a therapist present, although self-hypnosis is also an option in some cases. Generally, meditation involves directing focus either toward the body or away from it. When focused inward, a process known as mindfulness meditation, the patient tries to become more aware of his or her own body and in that way seize more control over functions that might otherwise be considered unconscious (heart rate, breathing). When focused outward, a process known as transcendental meditation, the patient instead tries to focus on some image or thought to the exclusion of all others, including pain. Meditation also has a great deal in common with biofeedback treatment, save that no external monitoring equipment is used. In fact, it might be possible to begin chronic pain treatment by using biofeedback equipment in a doctor's office before graduating to a meditative technique that can be performed anywhere.

Another alternative treatment method that has become increasingly popular in the last few years is chiropractic treatment. Chances are that your familiarity with chiropractors begins and ends with the image of someone twisting a patient's neck or spine until there's a cracking sound. Obviously, the practice doesn't literally involve breaking bones; that sound is created by escaping gas buildup between the vertebrae. The theory behind chiropractic treatment is that many of the health problems we suffer from can be traced back to misaligned posture. Now, while we can obviously see a connection between poor posture and back or neck pain, many of chiropractors other claims are viewed with a great deal of skepticism by the medical community. For instance, no medical evidence supports the claim that chiropractors can effectively treat Alzheimer's disease or cerebral palsy. On the other hand, an increasing number of physicians are open to referring their patients to chiropractors for issues connected with muscle mobilization and physical therapy.

Perhaps the most important lesson to learn from alternative treatment methods is that pain management is still a growing field of research. We are learning about new methods of pain management every year. At the same time, we're constantly reviewing old, once-discredited methods with an open mind. The biggest drawback to many of these treatments often comes from the practitioners themselves, who are sometimes inclined to credit alternative treatments as cure-alls for a host of conditions that they can in no way effectively treat. As always, it's important for you to clearly communicate with both your physician and any alternative treatment specialists, making sure to not only communicate your symptoms, but also to make sure that each knows what the other is telling you.

Physical Rehabilitation

The temptation when dealing with pain is to apply as little stress to the affected area as possible. While this is usually a wise course of action for short-term acute pain, it can lead to problems when dealing with long-term conditions. By now, it should be obvious that the "ignore it and it will go away" approach does not work when dealing with chronic pain. This is why, in addition to all of the other treatment methods we've already gone over, it's often vital to engage in physical rehabilitation. This is especially true if the patient has been avoiding treatment for an extended period of time, which can often exacerbate the problem of muscle damage by compounding it with muscle atrophy. Several forms of physical rehabilitation are worth exploring during treatment.

Physical therapy is perhaps the most basic and straightforward method of physical rehabilitation and involves the patient going through a guided series of activities for the purpose of increasing muscle strength and joint motion. These activities can include specific exercises, weight lifting, and stretching. Generally, patients will use physical therapy when recovering from an injury or surgery, but it's also been used for patients coping with cancer, arthritis, and a variety of other conditions that can limit movement. When choosing a physical therapist, you'll want to consider how much experience they have in dealing with your specific source of pain; there are, for example, physical therapists who specialize in arthritis, back pain, and physical rehabilitation after an accident.

Massage therapy may also be an option for the patient, especially in conjunction with more traditional physical therapy. A massage therapist will help to ease pain by physically manipulating muscles in the patient's body. This method can be especially helpful immediately after a physical therapy session, when the patient is feeling sore. As far as choosing a massage therapist goes, that will depend entirely on the type of pain being treated and what your doctor recommends. One form of massage, neuromuscular therapy massage, is specifically focused on alleviating chronic pain by focusing on muscular "trigger points," as well as overall posture and circulation issues. Other forms of massage include Shiatsu, deep tissue, Swedish, hot stone, Thai, and reflexology. There are massage therapists who specialize in each of these treatment methods, as well as in treating certain conditions, in much the same way as physical therapists. Despite the extensive training and state certification massage therapists undergo, it is important that you avoid turning to them for medical guidance.

For patients who lack the muscle strength to engage in physical therapy unaided, pool therapy might also be a viable option. Also known as water therapy and aquatic therapy, pool therapy involves performing a series of modified physical therapy exercises while submerged in a pool. Since the water supports a significant portion of the patient's weight, he or she feels a great deal less strain when moving. This type of therapy can be especially useful for patients suffering from muscle atrophy as they rebuild their strength.

The challenge with physical therapy, massage therapy, and pool therapy is that they tend to require the patient to show up regularly for appointments with a special therapist. Since it's not always possible to maintain such appointments and since there's only so much good that can come from meeting once or twice a week for an hour at a time, many doctors also recommend that patients maintain a regular home exercise routine in order to strengthen muscle tone, as well as to improve cardiovascular activity and a variety of other effects that can improve one's overall health.

Home exercise doesn't necessarily have to take place exclusively at home, and it's quite common for patients involved with pain management programs to join a fitness center. When joining a fitness center, it's obviously important that you speak with the staff members about any health issues you have, including pain management issues. Fortunately, many such centers have specialized exercise programs that target these issues. Special exercise styles like Pilates, a low-impact series of exercises meant to improve the strength of the abdomen, back, and hips, are becoming increasingly popular for individuals coping with a variety of conditions, including chronic pain.

As always, each new method added to the comprehensive pain management treatment plan can provide further relief and improved recovery for the patient. Many of these new methods will also require additional specialists (physical therapists, massage therapists, and fitness trainers) who need to be informed about a patient's medical conditions in order to provide the most effective treatment and avoid unintentionally causing damage by placing too much stress on parts of the body that are still recovering. As with each method we've covered, the obligation must fall to the patient to clearly communicate his or her symptoms with everyone involved in the pain management process.

The Future of Pain Management

My first exposure to chronic pain management was my grandmother's cancer pain. That was decades ago and half a world away. Looking over all of the pain treatment methods available to patients today, it can sometimes seem a bit overwhelming. And when I consider the unique challenges involved in making all of these diverse treatments work together, I'm glad that I don't have to do it alone. My patients are often treated by a team of specialists, each one handling a different aspect of the recovery process. With so much of the treatment depending on the patient's involvement, one of the most important tasks I perform is in providing them with a proper education concerning their options and responsibilities during treatment. And my patients aren't the only ones in need of further education, because as I stated earlier, pain management is a growing field of study.

Innovations are still being made in all five areas of comprehensive pain management. Pharmaceutical companies are constantly developing and testing new medications. Behavior modification methods are gaining more widespread acceptance among doctors, with equal support from health insurance providers. Interventional therapy continues to be developed so that it is both safer and less invasive. An increasing number of doctors are overcoming the long-held stigma against many alternative treatment methods, even as significant research is being conducted to better understand why these methods work. And physical therapy is one of the fastest growing career fields in the United States. With the baby boomer generation finally entering retirement age, the senior population is growing faster than ever, and with that growth comes an increase in individuals suffering from cancer, arthritis, nerve disease, and a variety of other conditions that bring with them chronic pain.

Unfortunately, the challenges facing both pain management specialists and those suffering from chronic pain have multiplied as well. Many of these challenges stem from the very growth of the pain management field, which invites further intervention from the government and various institutions — pharmaceutical companies, hospitals, and health insurance providers — to maintain accountability and profitability. There are also opportunists who see the chance to make money off the desperation of those dealing with chronic pain.

Health Care Costs

Health care costs have been steadily rising over the last few decades and likely will continue to rise for the foreseeable future. In the United States, the costs of health care are covered by a combination of private companies and government programs that provide health insurance. Whether or not this is the best possible system for health care management isn't a topic I'll be discussing here, since many experts have already written books defending every possible position on this issue. Rather, I'll focus on the system that is currently in place and the challenges that it presents to pain management specialists.

Quite simply, whenever government or private business is involved in a decision, there will be a demand (sooner or later) for results that are both tangible and easy to measure. If you're a building contractor, then your progress can be measured in how much of a building has been constructed, how many days it will take to finish constructing it, and how much money has been spent on materials and labor. In addition, a building will be inspected by various agencies for things as specific as the number of fire extinguishers on each floor, the width of the hallways, and the placement of various signs. These measures are conducted to maintain both profitability and safety. Chronic pain management is measured and evaluated using similar methods.

Unfortunately, pain management is not as easy to quantify as a house or office building. Pain is often a subjective experience that can't be accurately described. When you stub your toe in the shower, how do you measure the amount of pain you feel? When you burn your hand on a hot stove, how do you measure that amount of pain? If you break down the amount of pain from the stubbed toe into units, how many stubbed toe pain units would equal the pain of a burned hand? Now imagine having to keep a daily log of such pain units in order to measure their progress until you get back to zero, also taking into account that you'll have to subtract pain units you might be feeling due to illness, stress, and other injuries. Then imagine having to consult with another individual and somehow finding a way for him or her to confirm that the pain ratings you're giving are accurate. It's impossible . . . but it is the system that pain management specialists are expected to work in.

It's common for physicians to ask patients to rate their pain on a scale of one to ten (with one being mild and ten being unbearable), but this requires a level of objectivity from the patient that isn't always possible. Compare this to a cardiologist who can measure your heart rate down to a specific number of beats per minute. A phlebotomist can provide a chemical breakdown of every element and its percentage in a sample of your blood. Bone density, muscle-to-fat ratio, lung capacity, plaque build-up on teeth . . . all of these things can be measured accurately, and a second doctor can be called in to double-check the results and confirm them. But when a patient is asked to rate his or her own pain level, there is no way to double-check or confirm any of it. Not only does that make it difficult to estimate how much pain a patient is feeling, but it also makes it difficult to measure the effectiveness of treatment.

This lack of verifiable results is one of the reasons that so many forms of pain treatment are difficult to recommend. Insurance companies aren't going to pay out on treatments that don't seem to work, and if the only "evidence" presented is the patient picking a number between one and ten once a week and that number getting lower over several months, they may suspect that the whole thing is just a scam. There is no "pain meter" that can be attached to the patient's skin to provide an objective pain score. When doctors try to explain the complex nature of pain evaluation to insurance companies and government regulatory agencies, the sheer amount of information leads to confusion.

More complex scales have been developed, where an individual answers a whole series of questions to get a number, which equates patient level of pain or disability. Even though this may be a better solution, many patients get upset with the time it takes to fill out these questionnaires. Another thing that greatly hurts the reputation of genuine pain management techniques are all of the scams and hoaxes out there.

Hoaxes

Most medical hoaxes involve a "miracle" cure-all formula, something reassuringly all natural, yet also composed of mysteriously foreign ingredients. Various public figures would be rumored to have taken the cure, always to fantastic effect. All manner of medical authorities would be said to have endorsed the product, perhaps even with the proof of some signed documentation.

Flip through the channels on your television on any given night or simply type "miracle cure" into an Internet search engine, and you'll find videos that use all of the same tried and true methods. The cures are still "all natural." The pitches will often involve references to remedies that have been used in Asia or Europe for years, but until now have been kept out of the United States due to some vague conspiracy between doctors and pharmaceutical companies. The celebrity endorsement is also common, as it provides viewers with a common face to reassure them that the drug is safe and effective. As far as the medical endorsements go, that was never the key to an effective sales pitch, so it's usually little more than a passing reference to some medical study or other.

And when it comes to pain management, the miracle cures aren't limited to drugs. They can involve electrical devices, modified physical therapy equipment, or claims to the supernatural. Unfortunately, to many patients who have suffered for years from chronic pain, an epidural injection of anti-inflammatory medication may sound as plausible as someone using his magic powers to drive out pain demons. By using the power of suggestion, many patients can be convinced (at least temporarily) that these hoax cures are working. Again, the fact that pain is such a subjective topic means that it can be just as difficult to disprove the effectiveness of fake treatment as it is to prove the effectiveness of legitimate treatment.

Sadly, while many of the scam artists lead people to believe various fantastic claims about their treatments, they also tend to be careful about the specific wording of their claims so that, while misleading, they don't technically say anything that can be deemed untrue. For example, if I cited a study that said increased intake of calcium can help strengthen bones, that wouldn't mean that the calcium pills I was selling were a cure for bone cancer, but as long as I was careful to never explicitly say those things, I could talk about the studies, show a bunch of bone diagrams, and speak with people suffering from bone cancer, then let desperate viewers draw their own conclusions.

So how can someone tell the difference between a legitimate pain treatment plan and a scam? More to the point, how do my patients know that I'm not simply a scam artist with a medical degree? There are several warning signs that will tip you off quickly to a miracle cure being a hoax.

First of all, legitimate pain treatment specialists will never use words like "miracle" or "magic" to describe their treatments. They will never promise that all of your pain symptoms will vanish immediately or "overnight" or "within twenty-four hours." The treatments they offer will have a variety of studies to back up their effectiveness. They won't talk about the medical community as some shady organization that's "afraid to tell the truth" about their revolutionary treatment method. They won't hesitate to work with your insurance provider and will never insist on being paid in cash. They won't offer you a large volume of medication at a "discount price." And, perhaps most of all, they won't grow desperate when you mention seeking a second opinion.

I work within a massive community of specialists and spent years researching the vast amount of literature dedicated to pain management. If you have read this far into my book, you hopefully realize that I will have no problem explaining at length how various treatments work. While working with insurance companies and government regulatory agencies isn't my favorite part of the job, I always aim for transparency. I recommend a variety of treatments for my patients and have no "one size fits all" method for all of them. And if my patients want a second opinion, I am happy to have a second set of eyes review the same problem.

Unfortunately, one of the key words that hoax cures use to describe themselves, besides "miracle" and "magic," is "innovative." There are a number of fantastic innovations being made in pain management research and, by giving fake treatments the same names as these legitimate avenues of study, they make it even more difficult for legitimate researchers to receive the necessary funding to continue.

Studies in New Technology

Entire books have been written about emerging pain management methods, but I'd like to spend a little time with two of the most promising: stem cell research and platelet-rich plasma research.

Stem cells are the first cells that we develop at the moment we're conceived. If you've ever seen time-lapse photographs showing the week-by-week development of a fetus, you'll notice that at first it looks like nothing more than a pink ball. But eventually you begin to notice large features such as the head and limbs. The skin is transparent enough that you can see crude organs forming as well. The shift from pink ball to crude figure marks the shift when stem cells give way to bone cells, skin cells, and various other cells. What's important to remember is that those stem cells have the potential to become any number of other types of cells and merely await the proper chemical signals to determine what sort of cells they will become.

The theory that guides much of stem cell research is that if such stem cells are placed near damaged parts of a mature body, those chemical signals can be replicated and the stem cells will give way to new cells of the type needed. For example, in the future it may be possible to replace damaged nerve cells, such as in a broken spinal column, by stem cells that will eventually become new nerve cells. Stem cells can also be injected in damaged joints and ligaments, creating new tissue and replacing the damaged area that was the source of pain.

Stem cell research has encountered a number of challenges over the last few decades. As mentioned, there are scam artists who claim to employ stem cell technology and set up "clinics" where they will inject people with stem cell solutions. These solutions, of course, contain no such material, but even if they did, the injection method is usually so crude, using none of the technology outlined earlier to properly direct it, that it would do no good and possibly a great deal of harm. The other major problem is that many people object to the use of stem cell material due to misconceptions about how that material is acquired.

Another research method involves platelet-rich plasma. A platelet is a type of cell that's found in the blood. Its function is to recognize when the body has suffered damage and to bind blood cells together when that happens. Platelets are the reason your blood suddenly starts to clot after you've been cut. In addition, platelets send out signals when they recognize that the body has suffered some sort of damage, in order to draw in healing proteins. As far as pain treatment goes, platelet-rich plasma can be used to draw additional healing proteins to painful areas of the body that are not necessarily the result of an injury, such as an aching joint, in order to accelerate recovery.

The current technologies being used in pain management — using X-rays and ultrasound to direct injections, various new opioid and non-opioid pharmaceuticals — are still being improved upon as well, but it's reassuring to see new and seemingly unrelated technologies being employed in pain management. In the same way, we're learning more about pain management by devoting further study toward the patients themselves. In particular, there is one serious affliction that may provide clues to better treating pain symptoms.

Studies in Congenital Insensitivity to Pain

Congenital insensitivity to pain, CIP or congenital analgesia, as the name suggests, is a condition in which the patient is unable to feel pain or unable to respond to it. There are several causes for this condition, including a problem with NMDA (N-methyl-D-aspartate) receptors in the nerve endings. But the result is that an individual not only doesn't feel pain, but has never felt pain. Since pain often motivates self-preservation practices, infants and children are often especially in danger since there is no natural deterrent against activities that many of us avoid due to the pain it would cause — placing a hand in fire, touching sharp objects, falling. Since pain is also an early warning sign to various other health problems, individuals have to be extremely alert to other body signals throughout their lives.

While research is being conducted to treat this condition, there are also obvious benefits to being at least temporarily unable to experience pain. Research into what causes CIP could eventually lead to innovations in anesthesia and other pain relief methods. In the same manner, the research being done in various methods for alleviating pain might one day be used to treat CIP.

Conclusion

Maybe this book seems information heavy. But, in fact, it's little more than a primer for individuals suffering from chronic pain. Specialists in this field can devote decades to researching it and yet find that they still have so much left to learn. If anyone reading this book is suffering from a persistent pain, I would urge you to consult with a physician. "Toughing it out" and "waiting for it to go away" are not valid options.

At the same time, I encourage anyone dealing with chronic pain to do their own research. Keeping yourself informed is the best way to avoid hoaxes and scams. Don't be afraid to ask questions, and don't be afraid to seek a second opinion.

I still like the sound of rain. It reminds me of all the moments I spent as a boy with my grandma, listening to the raindrops fall on the windows as we both would talk about the past, the present, and even the future. Those memories I will always treasure. Though her future was cut short by breast cancer and she suffered in her final days, I'd like to think that she is somewhere smiling, knowing that we are entering a world of possibilities, a world where we can live pain free.

About The Author

Dr. Cassim is a board-certified physiatrist (PM&R) with additional certification in pain management from the American Board of Pain Medicine (ABPM). He earned his medical degree at NOVA Southeastern Medical School in Florida and completed his residency in Physical Medicine and Rehabilitation (PM&R) at the University of Minnesota where he served as chief resident. He continued on to complete his Pain and Interventional Management Fellowship training at the University of Minnesota, Riverside.

Dr. Cassim then worked in private practice in Minneapolis, MN, where he collaborated on a multidisciplinary team, treating a diverse group of pain conditions, focusing on spinal mediated pain. He specializes in interventional injection and implantable therapies for pain. He also worked as a primary and sub-investigator for Medical Applied Research Center (MARC) with patient centered research studies to help improve clinical treatment and outcomes related to pain.

Made in the USA
Lexington, KY
04 February 2017